Incredible Ways To CONTROL, IMPROVE, and REVERSE Your Diabetes

STEVEN DAVIS

CONTENTS

Introduction

I want to thank you and congratulate you for purchasing the book, *Incredible Ways To CONTROL, IMPROVE, And IMPROVE Your Diabetes.*

This book has actionable strategies on how to control diabetes.

Being diagnosed with diabetes may sound like a death sentence. However, this is not the case. Many people have lived long healthy lives even after being diagnosed with diabetes by simply changing their lifestyle. This, however, does not mean that adopting a new lifestyle is a piece of cake. It is definitely challenging but what other option do you have? Continue living an unhealthy life and die just a few years down the line? I know you would not want this or else you would not be reading this.

This book will help you understand more about diabetes, some amazing dieting, exercising and general tips to help you manage and control your diabetes so that you can live a normal, long and fulfilling life. Thanks again for purchasing this book, I hope you enjoy it!

Chapter 1: What Potential Causes and Who Usually Get Diabetes

Diabetes is a condition that is associated with too much blood glucose in your body such that the relevant mechanisms responsible for controlling these levels are unable to do that. This may be caused by your pancreas producing little or no insulin to help the cells in your body assimilate glucose or the insulin produced is inefficient (referred to as insulin resistance).

Insulin is a hormone that is secreted by the pancreas and facilitates the movement of glucose into the body's cells to be converted into energy so that you can work, play, and live your life. Glucose is usually broken down from carbohydrates and insulin helps in the absorption of glucose into the cells with the excess being stored in the liver as glycogen. High level of blood sugar level probably due to lack of adequate insulin or due to taking high carbohydrate meals that keep the sugar levels high then lead to diabetes. There are two types of diabetes: Type I, and Type II diabetes.

Who Usually Gets Type I Diabetes?

10% of all adults struggling with diabetes have type I diabetes, which is treated by insulin doses on a daily basis, taken through either an insulin pump or injections. Regular physical exercise and following a healthy diet are also recommended. There is usually no specific age at which type I diabetes can start, but most cases report it before the age of forty, and particularly in childhood. In fact, it is the most prevalent type of diabetes in children.

As earlier indicated, insulin is a hormone that serves as a chemical messenger to facilitate the conversion of glucose to energy in your blood. It is a sort of a key that opens the door to the cells in your body. Unlocking this door allows the glucose to enter the cells to be used as fuel. In case of type I diabetes, your body is unable to produce insulin, the door stays closed, and glucose accumulates in the blood. The body is unable to produce energy and tries to acquire glucose from somewhere else, leading to the breakdown of protein and fat stores instead. This can result in weight loss. Since the glucose is not being used by your body, it ends up being disposed in urine. Since you cannot live with such high levels of glucose, and you need the glucose since it is the fuel that our body runs on, you then need to take insulin doses in order to open the door for the cells to access nutrients to produce energy.

Who Usually Gets Type II Diabetes?

In case of type II diabetes, the pancreas fails to produce adequate insulin or the insulin produced is not effective (insulin resistance).

In most cases, diabetes type II appears in people over 40 years of age, although in South Asia, where it is highly prevalent, it usually occurs from the age of twenty-five. More and more cases are being reported in young people, adolescents, and children of all ethnicities. 85 to 95% of all diabetes cases are accounted for by type II diabetes, which is treatable with increased physical activity and a healthy diet. Insulin and medication are also often required. The insulin produced in Type II diabetes cases is usually insufficient or inefficient, which means that the cells are partially unlocked, leading to a slow buildup of glucose in your blood.

With that understanding of diabetes, let us now move on to some basics of diabetes once you know you have the condition.

The ABCs Of Diabetes

Consult your health care provider on how to manage your cholesterol, blood pressure, and A1C. This can go a long way towards reducing your risk of having a stroke, heart attack, or other diabetes complications.

A1C Test

This test calculates your overall blood sugar level for the past 3 months and is different from your daily blood sugar checks.

It is important to be familiar with your blood sugar levels with time. These numbers should not get too high, as high blood sugar levels can affect your eyes, feet, kidneys, blood vessels, and heart.

For most people with diabetes, the A1C goal is less than 7. However, this varies from person to person.

Blood Pressure

This is basically the force through which blood travels across your blood vessels.

High blood pressure is strenuous on your heart, and can lead to a stroke, heart attack, as well as damage to your eyes and kidneys. For most diabetics, the blood pressure should be less than 140/90, but this varies from person to person.

Cholesterol

Cholesterol comes in two forms: HDL and LDL.

LDL is the "bad" cholesterol that can accumulate in your blood and clog the blood vessels, leading to a stroke or a heart attack. On the other hand, HDL is the "good" cholesterol that helps to get rid of the "bad" cholesterol.

Chapter 2: Diabetes Dieting Tips and What Foods to Eat

Whether you are looking to control or prevent diabetes, you can make a significant difference by adjusting your lifestyle. One of the most significant steps you can take is to lose weight. The good news is that you don't have to shed off all those extra pounds in order to start experiencing the benefits. Studies have shown that losing just about 5 to 10 percent of your overall body weight can reduce your blood sugar substantially, in addition to lowering your cholesterol and blood pressure levels. Eating healthier and losing weight can also have a significant effect on your energy levels, mood, and a general sense of wellbeing.

It is never too late to incorporate positive changes in your life, even if you are already struggling with full-blown diabetes. Being overweight is the biggest risk factor for getting diabetes, but all body fat is designed differently. If most of your weight is centered around your abdomen, your risk is higher as opposed to if the fat is in your thighs and hips. But why is the risk higher with apple-shaped people than pear-shaped people?

Most of the fat in "pears" is stored below the skin, while that in "apples" is stored around the middle, majority of it find its way into the belly, circling their liver and abdominal organs. This type of fat has been closely associated with diabetes and insulin resistance.

Let us look at different ways of controlling and improving diabetes.

1. Slow Release, High Fiber Carbs

Carbohydrates are highly influential on your blood sugar levels as compared to proteins and fats, but it is not necessary to avoid them. You only have to be careful about the types of carbohydrates you consume. It is generally wise to restrict highly refined carbohydrates such as rice, pasta, and white bread, as well as snack foods, candy, and soda. Rather, concentrate on high fiber complex carbs, otherwise referred to as slow release carbohydrates. These help maintain normal blood sugar levels because they take a longer time to be digested, which automatically prevents your body from generating excess insulin. In addition, they provide longer lasting energy and keep you satisfied for longer.

Some of the fiber rich carbs you should consider include:

- Wild rice or brown rice

- Low sugar bran flakes

- Rolled oats or steel cut oats

- Low sugar, high fiber breakfast cereal

- Whole grain or whole wheat bread

- Whole wheat pasta

- Cauliflower, winter squash, yams, sweet potatoes

- Wild rice or brown rice

2. Simplify Glycemic Index and Easily Keep Track of Sugar Levels

The glycemic index refers to the speed with which food is converted into sugar in your body. Glycemic load, on the other hand, accounts for the amount of carbohydrate in a given food. Foods that have a high GI can spike your blood sugar significantly while those with a low GI have the least impact. There are several glycemic load and glycemic index tables available online, but you don't have to depend on food charts when trying to make wise choices. There is a simpler way to regulate the carbohydrates you take, which involves first classifying foods into 3 major categories: coal, water, and fire. It is generally better when your body has to work harder to break down food.

- *Coal foods*

These are rich in protein and fiber, with a low GI. They include beans, whole grains, seafood, lean meats, seeds, and nuts, in addition to "white food" substitutes such as whole-wheat pasta, whole-wheat bread, and brown rice.

- *Water foods*

These are free foods, which mean that they can be eaten as much as you desire. They include most types of fruit and all vegetables.

- *Fire foods*

These are low in protein and fiber, with a high GI. They include chips, sweets, "white foods" (most baked foods, potatoes, white bread, white pasta, and white rice), as well as many processed foods. You should limit these in your diet.

3. Control Weight With Glycemic Index

Studies have shown that the key to controlling weight lies in limiting the amount of refined carbohydrates in your diet (the "fire" or "white" foods), and concentrating on the "coal" or low GI foods that keep you feeling satisfied for longer. Foods that have a low glycemic index are digested slower, so sugar takes more time to be absorbed into your bloodstream. This subsequently reduces your chances of experiencing a spike in blood sugar levels, keeps you feeling fuller for longer and makes you less likely to overeat.

Go for whole fresh fruit as opposed to fruit juice.

*Avoid processed foods such as packaged cereal, sugary desserts, and baked foods, and instead choose whole grains, dark green leafy vegetables, fat-free low sugar yogurt, beans, and steel cut oats.

4. Wise Choices on Sugar Intake

While you don't have to eliminate sugar altogether when you are struggling with diabetes, chances are you take more sugar than you are supposed to.

If you have a sweet tooth, you'll be interested to know that it is possible to eliminate cravings and change preferences while still enjoying a small serving of your preferred dessert.

*Combine sweets with a meal, as opposed to singular snacks: Desserts and sweets can spike your blood sugar when consumed on their own. You can control your blood sugar by combining them with other healthy foods especially foods high in fiber.

*Incorporate some healthy fat in your dessert: Choosing higher fat desserts against their fat free or low-fat counterparts may seem counterintuitive, but fat puts a break on the digestive process, thus preventing blood sugar levels from spiking rapidly. However, avoid the donuts and go for healthy fats such as yogurt, ricotta cheese, peanut butter, or some nuts.

5. Alcohol Intake Levels

It can be easy to underestimate the amount of carbohydrates and calories contained in alcoholic drinks, including wine and beer. In addition, cocktails blended with juice and soda can be packed with sugar. If it is necessary to drink, do it in moderation (at most 2 drinks per day for men, and one drink for women). Combine your drink with food, and go for calorie-free drink choices. Monitor your blood glucose consistently, since alcohol can impede on insulin and diabetes medication.

Reduce the amount of juice, soda, and soft drinks you take. A certain study revealed that for every 12-ounce sugar-sweetened beverage you take every day, you increase your risk for diabetes by approximately fifteen percent. If you need a carbonation kick, go for sparkling water with a squeeze of lime or lemon, or a splash of fresh fruit juice. Also, avoid adding sweeteners and creamers to your coffee and tea beverages.

Sugar is also concealed in many fast food meals, packaged foods, and grocery store staples like ketchup, low fat meals, frozen dinners, instant mashed potatoes, margarine, pasta sauce, canned soups & vegetables, sweet drinks, cereals, and bread. Therefore, be cautious when buying food.

6. Choosing Fats

Generally, fats are either bad or good. A study that followed 27,000 people who were between the ages of 45-74 for 14 years showed that those who ate healthy fats like olive oil reduced their risk of diabetes by 25%. This shows that healthy fats are actually good for you. However, all fats are rich in calories; therefore, take them in moderation. Below are the good and unhealthy fats.

Healthy fats: These are unsaturated fats, whose sources are fish and plants, and are basically liquid at room temperature. The main sources include avocados, nuts, canola oil, and olive oil. Concentrate on omega 3 fatty acids as well, which support heart and brain health, and fight inflammation. You can find these in flaxseeds, tuna, and salmon.

Unhealthy fats: Trans fats and saturated fats are the most destructive fats. Saturated fats originate from animal products like red meat, as well as whole milk dairy products. On the other hand, trans fats (aka partially hydrogenated oils) are made by blending vegetable oils with hydrogen in order to solidify them.

7. Perfect Usage of Vinegar on Meals

Are you aware that a spoonful of vinegar can actually lower your blood sugar levels? Simply adding a tablespoon or two to your meal can help reduce the post-meal increase in blood glucose by around 40%. This is because vinegar can inhibit digestion of starch and hold it in the stomach for just a little longer; thus, reducing chances of sugar spikes. This, however, does not mean you go crazy on carbs then add vinegar.

8. Eat Regularly Within Your Schedule

As said at the beginning, you don't have to lose all your excess weight when struggling with diabetes in order to reap all the benefits. What's more, you don't have to starve yourself or obsessively count your calories. Studies have shown that eating regularly and journaling what you eat are two of the most effective strategies to lose weight. Your body is more capable of regulating your weight and blood sugar levels when you stick to a regular meal schedule. Go for moderate, but consistent portion sizes for every snack or meal.

Do not skip breakfast: Take a good breakfast in the morning to start your day off. This will provide you with enough energy to tackle the better part of the day, and ensure steady blood sugar levels.

Maintain the same calorie intake: Being in control of the number of calories you take on a daily basis can affect the consistency of your blood sugar levels. Maintain the same number of calories each day, instead of not eating much one day, and then overeating on the next.

Eat small, regular meals: People have a tendency to overeat when they are very hungry, so taking regular meals will help you keep an eye on your portions. Furthermore, you don't want instances where your blood sugar goes really low then after a meal goes up too high. When you eat regular small meals, you are able to manage your sugar levels easily.

Keeping a food diary has been shown to be highly advantageous when you are trying to lose weight as well as monitor what triggers your high blood sugar levels. This is because it enables you to identify problem areas, for example, your morning latte or afternoon snack, where there are more calories than expected. What's more, it makes you more aware of what you are eating, how much, and why, which can help you cut back on emotional eating and mindless snacking.

Chapter 3: Easy and Simple Exercise For Diabetes

Before we look at the different kinds of exercises that you can try, it is important to understand the connection between exercise and diabetes and why it is important to exercise to control and improve your diabetes.

For starters, exercising makes it easier to control your blood sugar levels. As earlier indicated, when you have diabetes, you have a lot of glucose in your blood because either your body cannot produce insulin or because it does not use insulin properly. In both cases, exercise helps to reduce your blood glucose levels. This is because when exercising, your muscles need glucose, and since it is readily available in your blood, the muscles use the glucose they need and your glucose levels go down.

Secondly, if you have diabetes, you are likely to develop other long-term complications like heart problems. Exercise is great because it makes your heart healthy and store and helps you lower bad cholesterol; hence avoiding arteriosclerosis.

Because you can start on your exercises, it is important to note as I have stated earlier that if you have, you are at an increased risk of developing coronary artery disease. If you are 35 years old and above and are looking to start a moderate to high-intensity exercise regimen, it is advisable to undertake screening for cardiovascular disease. In addition, if you are 25 years of age or older, and have had type II diabetes for more than ten years, or type I diabetes for more than fifteen years, you should be screened as well. Since some activities can cause detached retina or retinal hemorrhage in the location of proliferative retinopathy, it is recommended that you consult with your ophthalmologist before starting an exercise program.

If you are a type I diabetic, you should tailor your exercise regimen to your specific condition. For example, if you have peripheral neuropathy, you should be careful to avoid abrasions and blisters, and be watchful of such conditions after working out. Consider delaying your exercise if your blood glucose is more than 250ml/dl, with the presence of ketones, or if your blood glucose level is greater than 300mg/dl.

You should monitor your blood glucose before, during, and after working out, and take precautions against hypoglycemia, which can occur several hours after or even during exercise. Ensure you have some carbohydrates at hand, and take them as needed to avoid hypoglycemia.

Assessing Exercise Risks

Increasing your physical activity comes with its own risks when you are struggling with diabetes. However, being sedentary is much worse

– it does not contribute to your wellbeing, diabetes management, weight management, or glucose control. To minimize potential risks and reap the benefits of enhanced physical activity, you need to be familiar with and evaluate the risks involved in advance, and then take the necessary steps to prevent them before they occur.

Hypoglycemia

Hypoglycemia is a major concern for diabetics who are under insulin or any medication. Your muscles use glucose whenever you engage in physical activity. They start by gobbling up the glucose stored as glycogen, after which glucose pours from the blood to your muscles to cater for their energy requirements, subsequently reducing blood glucose levels. Your body needs to refill the glucose storage containers of its muscles to prepare for further movement. This can lead to a hypoglycemic reaction during both periods of physical activity and several hours later. If you tend to experience hypoglycemia frequently, it may be easy to associate any form of physical activity with an imbalance in glucose control. In this case, failure to conduct glucose testing can keep you in the dark about your body's reaction to activity. This in turn makes you unprepared for the reduced blood glucose level, which may happen when you mow the lawn, or simply take a brisk stroll around the park. You may resort to taking a handful of jelly beans to counter the low, with the result of skyrocketing your glucose level. So you take extra medication or insulin during dinner to counter the high, only to find your blood glucose fluctuation continuing with another drop before you go to bed.

This roller coaster ride can lead to a great deal of frustration and confusion, leaving you scared and upset. If you are struggling with this scenario, it can be beneficial to increase your blood glucose testing to better understand your body's reaction to exercise, and be prepared.

Heart Disease

As said previously, people with diabetes have an increased risk of developing coronary heart disease. As such, it is important to consult with your doctor before proceeding with any kind of physical activity and conduct an exercise intolerance test if necessary. This test is carried out on a treadmill and evaluates your heart's strength to function under stress. Regardless of the outcome of the test, chances are you can still be able to engage in physical activity.

Diabetes Complications

As a general rule of thumb, it is advisable to account for any possible related conditions or diabetic complications before increasing your level of activity. People with particular medical conditions may not be compatible with certain types of activity. For instance, if you are dealing with hypertension, any exercise that includes straining, like weight lifting, can significantly increase your blood pressure during the workout, and aggravate the condition even further.

To limit any possible complications, you need to control your blood pressure well before engaging in any level of activity, especially those that involve straining. Straining can also aggravate proliferative retinopathy, which raises the pressure within some weakened blood vessels in the eyes. Acute hemorrhage can also develop in weakened eye vessels when you engage in activities that involve rapid head motions or jarring or require straining. As such, it is important to conduct an eye check for retinopathy signs before embracing an exercise regimen and have them checked again annually. If you are suffering from substantial nerve disease in the feet, it may be difficult to feel injuries in your feet, most of which are blisters. However, this does not mean that you should not exercise. It only means that you should consult your doctor first, and observe proper foot care while at home. It may also come in handy asking for expert advice on the right footwear for the particular activity, and ensure that the chosen footwear matches your feet. Here are the best exercises to help you get started in your journey to manage and control diabetes:

- **Walking**

Since walking can be done by anyone in almost any place, and it is less strenuous, it is the most common and highly recommended exercise for people dealing with diabetes. Start with 30 minutes to 1 hour of brisk walking, 3 times per week.

- **Practicing Tai Chi**

This type of exercise originated from the Chinese and uses gentle and smooth body movements to calm the body and mind. The exercise has been shown to improve blood sugar control significantly, as well as increase mental health, energy, and vitality.

- **Yoga**

This is a traditional form of exercise that uses fluid movements to increase balance, strength, and flexibility. It is beneficial for people struggling with various chronic conditions, like diabetes. This is because it improves nerve function and lowers stress levels, which subsequently results in increased wellness and state of mental health. The reason why yoga helps improve blood glucose levels has been linked to improved muscle mass.

- **Dancing**

Dancing can do wonders for your body. The psychological work involved to remember dance sequences and steps can actually improve your memory and boost your brain power. If you are struggling with diabetes, it can be a fun way to increase your physical activity, reduce stress, lower blood sugar, improve flexibility, and promote weight loss. There is even chair dancing that involves the use of a chair to dance for people with physical disabilities. A mere thirty minutes of dancing can burn up to one hundred and fifty calories for a 150-pound person.

- **Swimming**

Swimming expands and contracts your muscles, without straining your joints. If you are struggling with diabetes, it can help lower stress levels, burn calories, and improve cholesterol levels. For the best results, it is recommendable to swim for at least 10 minutes, three times per week, gradually increasing the length of your workout. Be sure to monitor your blood sugars and have a snack. In addition, be sure to inform the lifeguard that you are dealing with diabetes before getting into the pool.

Here are some super effective tips to help with your exercise:

Quick Workouts

As long as your total workout sums up to thirty minutes every day, several brief exercises are fine. People with diabetes need to be up and moving – if you can stretch your exercise into one thirty minute session, cool; otherwise, break it into manageable increments that'll add up to thirty minutes of exercise per day. Remember you don't want your sugar levels to go really down and this is what is likely to happen if you do intense exercise for a long time.

Concentrate Activity

Increase your physical activity on a general basis; for example, climbing or walking, instead of a particular type of workout. However, avoid relying on housework or daily activities as the only exercise. It can be easy to underestimate the number of calories you consume and the amount of exercise you get.

Exercising With a Friend

Exercising can be very hard if you do not have anyone to encourage you, or you can easily get lonely exercising alone, and this can make you forget about exercising altogether. In order to be accountable and ensure you exercise as you have seen the benefits of exercising if you are diabetic, it is advisable to find someone to exercise with. It is actually better to exercise with someone else who is diabetic who understand what you may be going though as you exercise. You will not feel as though the person does not understand you when they scorn you because they have been through there and just as they are able to exercise so can you.

Avoid Glucose Complications

There are several things you can do to avoid complications with your glucose levels when exercising:

- If you use insulin to manage your diabetes, familiarize yourself with your insulin's peak time, and schedule your activities accordingly. When you avoid the peak and strongest times of your insulin, it will help you avoid hypoglycemia.

- If you are prone to hypoglycemia, be prepared for a probable hypoglycemic episode. Have glucose tablets all the time. In case you sense signs of low blood sugar, stop what you are doing immediately and take the quick acting glucose.

- Monitor your blood glucose thirty minutes before exercise, and just before, you start. This will give you a general idea of where your glucose level is directed, and plan for a low in advance.

- Schedule your activity to come after a meal in order to help reduce the accelerated blood glucose level, which follows eating.

- If you are planning to engage in an intense activity, check your glucose level right before you get started. If the level of your blood glucose is close to normal, but you are at a risk of developing hypoglycemia, it might be necessary to eat before the activity.

- Do not inject insulin on the muscle areas you are going to use during exercise. For instance, if it is tennis, avoid injecting the insulin on the racket arm, and perhaps even your legs. The buttocks or the abdomen are usually the best before an activity.

- If you check your blood glucose prior to the activity and find it to be >250mg/dl, check for ketones in your urine. If present, your blood glucose level may actually increase. Positive ketones and an elevated glucose level are an indication that your diabetes is out of order, and you need to consult your diabetes health care team right away.

- If, during an exercise, you happen to experience leg cramps, chest pain, or shortness of breath that disappear after resting, consult your doctor right away. All of these are possible symptoms of blocked arteries.

- Make sure that you take plenty of fluids. Sweat is a sign that you are excreting fluids, which need to be replaced. It is a good idea to have water by your side at all times.

- If you consistently experience hypoglycemic episodes during or after increased activity levels, consult your doctor and consider changing your medications.

Increasing your activity levels needs to be fun, or else you are less likely to make an active lifestyle last. Select your exercises accordingly, and participate in a little physical activity every day.

Chapter 4: Best Health Supplements for Diabetes

One of the main reasons why nutritional support is crucial is because diabetes is a condition that tends to waste and deplete nutrition. Hiked blood glucose levels behave like a diuretic, leading to significant loss of nutrients through the urine. As such, if you are struggling with diabetes, you are more likely to have a deficiency of vital water-soluble minerals and vitamins. Surprisingly, most professionals who specialize in diabetes do not attempt to replace the lost nutrients, and the patients end up paying the inevitable costs of nutritional deficiencies.

The second reason why it is essential to take nutritional supplements for diabetes is that increasing your nutrient intake carefully to enhance your body's ability to utilize insulin can go a long way towards maintaining healthy levels of your blood sugar. If you have diabetes, you should at least take a high-quality mineral and vitamin supplement every day.

Must Have Supplements For Reversing Diabetes

Ensure that you are getting the nutrients outlined below, besides a multivitamin. Several are incorporated into multivitamins, but sometimes not at the recommended dosages.

B-complex vitamins

Specifically, vitamins B12 and B6 support nerve health that is crucial for dealing with such conditions as diabetic neuropathy. Another vital

B complex vitamin is biotin, which is necessary for growth and metabolism. Biotin also plays a role in the production and utilization of carbohydrates, fats, and protein. Take 300mcg of biotin, 150mcg of B12, and 75mg of B6 every day.

Vitamin C

This supplement reduces sorbitol levels, the sugar that tends to accumulate in and damage cells in your nerves, kidneys, and eyes. The daily-recommended dose is 1,000 mg at the very least.

Vitamin D

Vitamin D stimulates genes that boost the manufacture of antimicrobial peptides referred to as cathelicidins, which terminate bacteria, viruses, and other germs. Since people with diabetes have a higher risk of developing infections due to periodontal disease and diabetic ulcers, it is important to ensure that your body has ideal levels of vitamin D. The daily-recommended dose of supplemental vitamin D is 2,000 IU at the very least.

Vitamin E

This is the best fat-soluble antioxidant for your body. It supports glucose control, and shields nerves and blood vessels from the damage of free radicals, which is fast-tracked by diabetes. In fact, high intake of supplemental vitamin E has been shown to reverse the damage caused by diabetes on the nerves, as well as protect against atherosclerosis, and diabetic cataracts. The daily-recommended dose for vitamin E is 300 IU at the very least, regardless of your health status.

However, ensure that you take the natural form of vitamin E only, which is usually listed as d-alpha-tocopheryl or d-alpha-tocopherol. You can differentiate it from synthetic vitamin E, which is usually listed as dl-alpha tocopheryl or dl-alpha-tocopherol.

Magnesium

This mineral is crucial for protein synthesis and energy production, DNA production, and cellular replication. Studies have also shown that magnesium can also help reduce insulin resistance. The daily-recommended dose is 500 to 1,000 mg every day.

Vanadium

Vanadium acts as insulin in your body and helps stabilize blood sugar levels. The daily-recommended dose is 100 mg.

Chromium

This trace mineral enhances the activity of insulin and helps transfer glucose into the cells, as well as other nutrients. Chromium does not facilitate the production of more insulin in your body – rather, it improves its efficiency. This mineral has also been shown to improve glucose metabolism. The daily recommended dose is 200mcg.

Berberine

This is a plant alkaloid whose target is AMPK (AMP-activated protein kinase), an ancient and very basic metabolism regulator that is present in all plants and animals. AMPK facilitates the absorption of glucose into your body's cells, reduces the production of glucose in your liver, and improves insulin sensitivity. The daily-recommended dose is 1,500mg.

Purslane

This is a plant that is generally considered to be a weed in America but enjoyed as a food in Asia and Europe. But purslane can also help control blood sugar levels. Research has shown that a patented extract of the plant can increase insulin sensitivity, slow the movement of glucose into the blood from the intestines, and enhance the uptake of glucose into the cells. The daily-recommended dose is 180mg.

Gymnema sylvestre

This is an extract of the leaves from a climbing plant that is native to the South and Central Indian forests. The leaves are packed with gymnemic acids, which can slow the transfer of glucose from the intestines into your blood. This subsequently helps maintain healthy levels of blood sugar. The daily-recommended dose is 200mg. You can also take 400mg for extra support.

Banaba leaf extract

This originated from Asia and is packed with colosolic acid, which promotes the transport of glucose into the cells, maintaining an even level of blood sugar in the process. The daily recommended dose is

3mg.

Herbs can have strong medicinal effects on your body, and interact

dangerously with some drugs. If you are under any medication,

consult with your doctor before embracing herbal products.

Chapter 5: Managing and Controling Diabetes

Stress, for people with diabetes, can interfere with blood glucose

levels in a number of ways. For starters, if you are stressed, you are

less likely to take care of yourself, and may even resort to alcohol, not

exercising, and an unhealthy diet. Secondly, stress hormones can have

a direct impact on your blood glucose levels.

Treatments for depression or anxiety, as well as stress management are all very significant parts in the treatment of diabetes. It can be easy to overlook these factors as you concentrate excessively on the exercise, food, and medications. However, too much stress in the background can directly aggravate your blood sugars.

To manage or reduce stress, it is advisable to engage in guided imagery biofeedback, meditation, exercise, listening to relaxing music, or simply reading a book. If your diabetes is one of the reasons why you are under stress, you may want to join a support group. Being familiar with other people in the same boat can help reduce the feeling of loneliness. In addition, they can provide helpful insights on how they cope with their own problems.

Dental, Skin, Foot, and Eye Care

It is vital that you schedule regular dental and eye appointments, and to monitor your skin and feet for diabetes-related complications such as dryness or sores. This is because diabetes affects the smallest blood vessels in your body, which are commonly found in your nerves, kidneys, and eyes. If you have diabetes, you are at a higher risk of glaucoma, cataracts, and blindness, but you can reduce your risk by managing your glucose levels. In addition, detecting and treating eye problems early can actually save your sight.

Being diabetic also means that you are at an increased risk of having gum complications since poor control of blood glucose increases the chances of gum problems. Standard dental hygiene practices like regular dental visits, daily flossing, and brushing your teeth twice every day can help avoid complications.

Approximately half of all diabetics are affected with some form of neuropathy or nerve damage, which can make you numb. This can, in turn, make you unresponsive to pain and other issues, particularly on your feet. As such, you can walk a distance with a sore on your foot, and this is what causes infections and, inevitably, amputations. Inspecting your feet regularly will come in handy. What's more, the nerves in your feet and legs may not receive the message to perspire, which is required to keep your skin moist and soft.

Why Flu Shots Matters

If suffering from diabetes, you are prone to having complication is you get the flu. You may even end up being hospitalized because of the flu. In addition, the flu can actually cause your blood sugar levels to increase drastically, and this can cause severe complications and make it hard for you to heal fast. This is because when you have the flu, as the body tries to fight the infection, the blood sugar levels rise, presenting a huge challenge for you. Therefore, make sure you get your flu shot each year.

Does Smoking Effect Diabetes?

I know quitting smoking is challenging. However, there is no any other way you can look at your situation. If you want to manage diabetes better, then quitting smoking should be top on your to-do things. Smoking increases insulin resistance and even narrows blood vessels, which can then interfere with circulation to your legs, and this can cause other complications. Since quitting completely may be hard, you can try to reduce how many cigarettes you smoke daily until a time when you no longer smoke.

Conclusion

Thank you again for purchasing this book!

I hope this book was able to help you to control and better manage diabetes.

The next step is to first determine where you are now and start changing your diet to improve your diabetes.

Thank you and good luck!

– Steven Davis

www.ingramcontent.com/pod-product-compliance
Lightning Source LLC
Chambersburg PA
CBHW071258280526
45788CB00004B/1759